Dash Diet

A Complete Beginner's Guide

Disclaimer

The ideas, concepts and opinions expressed in this book are intended to be used for educational purposes only. This book is provided with the understanding that the author and publisher are not rendering medical advice of any kind, nor is this book intended to replace medical advice, nor to diagnose, prescribe or treat any disease, condition, illness or injury.

It is imperative that before beginning any diet or exercise program, you receive full medical clearance from a licensed physician. Both the author and publisher claim no responsibility to any person or entity for any liability, loss, or damage caused or alleged to be caused directly or indirectly as a result of the use, application or interpretation of the material in this book.

A Quick Preview

We are what we eat! If we develop diseases due to eating unhealthy food, then logically we should get healthier once we start eating healthy food. That theory is actually true as proven by numerous studies conducted worldwide on the DASH diet! This relatively simple concept has evolved into the DASH diet, which helps significantly lower not only blood pressure but also provides powerful results for a whole lot of other diseases and ailments.

In this beginner's guide, you will learn everything you need to know about the DASH diet, including:

- What is DASH diet and why is it so popular?

- Health benefits of DASH diet

- Foods allowed on DASH diet

- A guide to planning your meals

- DASH exercise guide

- DASH breakfast, lunch, dinner, snacks and dessert recipes

Finally before bidding you good bye and good luck, we will share with you great tips on following DASH diet successfully.

Contents

Disclaimer 2

A Quick Preview 3

What is the DASH DIET? 7

Health benefits of DASH Diet 8

DASH Diet Food List 9

    Allowed Meats 9

    Allowed Grains 9

    Allowed Dairy Products (One Percent Fat or Fat Free) 10

    Allowed Nuts and Seeds 10

    Allowed Vegetables 10

    Allowed Oils and Fat 12

    Allowed Sugars 13

    Serving Sizes 14

        Size of 1 Serving of the Allowed Sugars 14

        Size of 1 Serving of the Allowed Meats 14

        Size of 1 Serving of the Allowed Fruits 14

        Size of 1 Serving of the Allowed Vegetables 14

        Size of 1 Serving of the Allowed Nuts and Seeds 14

        Size of 1 Serving of the Allowed Dairy 15

        Size of 1 Serving of the Allowed Grains 15

How to Plan Your Dash Diet 16

    Calculate Your Caloric Need 16

    What Should Those Calories Be Comprised of? 17

DASH Diet Exercise Routine 18

DASH Diet Breakfast Recipes 19

Go Green Smoothie 19

Nutritious Breakfast Pudding 20

Very Berry Smoothie 22

Power Packed Pancakes 23

Healthy Oat Bread 25

Peanut Butter Smoothie 27

French toast 28

DASH Diet Lunch 29

Tuna Salad 29

DASH Pizza 30

Pasta Salad 31

Salad Skewers 32

Strawberry Salad 33

Walnut Salad 35

Wild Salad 36

Flavored Yogurt Cups 37

Turkey Wraps 38

DASH Snacks 39

Apple Muffins 39

DASH Dip 41

DASH Blueberry Muffins 42

Paradise in a Cup Smoothie 44

DASH Hummus 45

Oat Muffins 46

Lemon Buttermilk 48

DASH Dinner 49

Chicken Dinner 49

Beef in Grilled Pineapple 51

Sausage and Beans 53

Tangy Halibut 54

Chili Stir Fry 55

Orange Chicken 56

DASH Dessert 58

Cocoa Pudding 58

Walnut and Chocolate Cookies 59

Popsicles 61

Blackberry Mock 62

Berry Crumble 63

Quick and Healthy Trifle 64

DASH Diet & Day Meal Planner 65

Crucial DASH Diet Tips 66

What is the DASH DIET?

The DASH Diet has recently been claimed to be the best diet of all, by doctors. The DASH diet stands for 'Dietary Approaches To Hypertension', and it was developed by the Nutritionist Marla Heller. Even though it has become widely popular due to its weight loss causing benefits, it was not originally created for this purpose.

As the name suggests, this diet is for people who want to reduce their blood pressure levels. However, due to the incredible weight loss effects, this diet has been used by many people, all over the world, who don't suffer from hypertension.

The purpose behind creating the DASH diet was to find a way to lower blood pressure without the use of medication. Various recent studies have proven that DASH diet is not only ideal for patients suffering from blood pressure related issues, but for anyone who wants to live a healthy, ailment free life.

According to health experts, a person should not consume more than twenty three hundred milligrams (2,300 mg) of sodium per day. However for those suffering from hypertension, the recommended amount is reduced to fifteen hundred milligrams (1,500 mg) of sodium intake daily. The relationship between the amounts of sodium in one's daily diet is directly proportional to the blood pressure level in a person's blood. As a result, by reducing the levels of sodium in one's diet, blood pressure can be brought down as well.

In numerous studies, it has been observed that on an average a US adult consumes approximately 4,200 milligrams of sodium daily; which is an extremely dangerous level of sodium. These findings also indicate that a vast population of people are on the path to easily developing this disorder if they don't reduce their daily sodium intake immediately. Keeping this fact in mind, the DASH menu contains exactly this amount of daily sodium intake, in order to maintain and reduce blood pressure levels.

Health benefits of DASH Diet

In the studies conducted on the DASH diet, a surprising effect was noticed in the people following the diet. It was observed that these people started gradually dropping pounds and reducing inches on their waists. As a result of this benefit, people have been religiously following the DASH diet and dropping their unwanted pounds and feeling better than ever. Along with weight loss, the research showed some other surprising benefits in people following the diet. These included:

1. Lowered blood pressure levels

2. Lowered blood cholesterol levels

3. Reduction in the risk of developing cancer

4. Lowered risk of developing chronic diseases

5. Reduction in blood sugar levels

6. Improved kidney health

DASH Diet Food List

Seeing the benefits of following the DASH diet, the first question that people usually ask is about the food items allowed in this diet. For your ease, we are listing the foods allowed on DASH diet, below. However you will be allotted specific serving sizes of food as per your required daily calorie consumption, which we will discuss in the next chapter.

Allowed Meats

1. Lean Fish and Chicken

2. Skinless Meat Cooked in a Healthy Way, such as by broiling, grilling, baking or boiling it

Allowed Grains

1. Bread

2. Dry cereals

3. Brown rice

4. Whole wheat pasta

5. Pita bread

6. Whole wheat bagels

7. Oatmeal

8. Unsalted pretzels

9. Brown rice

10. Butter free, unsalted popcorn

Allowed Dairy Products (One Percent Fat or Fat Free)

1. Milk

2. Yogurt

3. Cheese

4. Buttermilk

Allowed Nuts and Seeds

1. Peanuts

2. Walnuts

3. Almonds

4. Pistachios

5. Hazelnuts

6. Mixed nuts

7. Sunflower seeds

8. Peanut butter

9. Almond butter

10. Any nut butter

Allowed Vegetables

1. Broccoli

2. Carrots

3. Collards

4. Green beans

5. Green peas

6. Kale

7. Lettuce Leaves

8. Lima beans

9. Potatoes

10. Spinach

11. Squash

12. Sweet potatoes

13. Tomatoes

Allows Fruits

1. Grapes

2. Oranges

3. Apples

4. Dates

5. Grapefruit

6. Grapefruit Juice

7. Apricots

8. Bananas

9. Oranges

10. Orange Juice

11. Mangoes

12. Strawberries

13. Peaches

14. Sweet Melon

15. Watermelon

16. Pineapples

17. Papaya

Allowed Oils and Fat

1. Vegetable Oil

2. Olive Oil

3. Canola Oil

4. Corn Oil

5. Safflower Oil

6. Soft margarine

7. Low fat mayonnaise

8. Fat free salad dressing

Allowed Sugars

1. Sugar

2. Sorbet

3. Fruit Jelly

4. Sugar free candy

5. Sugar free fruit punch

6. Maple syrup

7. Fruit flavored gelatin

Serving Sizes

Size of 1 Serving of the Allowed Sugars

Sugar - 1 tablespoon

Sorbet - Half cup

Sugar free fruit jelly/ jam - Half cup

Lemonade - 1 cup

Size of 1 Serving of the Allowed Meats

Cooked meat - 1 ounce

Egg - 1

Size of 1 Serving of the Allowed Fruits

Fresh fruit - 1

Fruit juice - Half cup

Dried fruit - One-fourth cup

Sliced or diced fruit - Half cup

Size of 1 Serving of the Allowed Vegetables

Raw vegetables - 1 cup

Juiced vegetables - Half cup

Cooked vegetables - Half cup

Size of 1 Serving of the Allowed Nuts and Seeds

Nuts - One-third cup

Seeds - Half ounce

Peanut butter - 2 tablespoons

Cooked legumes, beans and peas - Half cup

Size of 1 Serving of the Allowed Dairy

Milk or yogurt - 1 cup

Cheese - 1½ ounces

Size of 1 Serving of the Allowed Grains

Bread - 1 slice

Cereals - 1 ounce

Cooked rice or pasta - Half cup

How to Plan Your Dash Diet

At first glance, the DASH diet may look a little complicated, what with all the serving sizes and allowed foods, but in the next step you will understand the link and as a result, the whole process will become much clearer.

Calculate Your Caloric Need

Age in Years	Daily Caloric Requirement For Women According to Daily Activity Level		
	Sedentary	Moderate	Active
19 - 30	2,000	2,200	2,400
31 - 50	1,800	2,000	2,200
Above 50	1,600	1,800	2,000

Every person's daily resting metabolic rate differs depending on their daily activity level. As a result, to calculate daily caloric requirement, it is necessary to take into account your daily activity levels. Take a look at the above table and based on your activity level, select your daily caloric requirement.

Age in Years	Daily Caloric Requirement For Men According to Daily Activity Level		
	Sedentary	Moderate	Active
19 - 30	2,400	2,800	3,000
31 - 50	2,200	2,600	2,800
Above 50	2,000	2,400	2,600

What Should Those Calories Be Comprised of?

Now that you know how many calories you are allowed to eat in a day based on your gender, the next step is to figure out how much you are allowed to eat from each of the food groups.

Food Category	Servings per Day Based on Daily Caloric Requirement				
	1,600	1,800	2,000	2,600	3,000
Grains	6	6	8	11	13
Vegetables	4	5	5	6	6
Fruits	4	5	5	6	6
Fat-free or low fat milk and milk products	2	2	3	3	4
Lean meats, poultry, and fish	5	6	7	7	9
Nuts, seeds, and legumes	3	4	5	1	1
Sugars	3	5	5	3	3

As you can see on this table, it has serving sizes of each food group based on the daily caloric requirement you calculated in the last table. If you are allowed 1,800 calories daily, looking at the table we can see that, you are allowed to eat 6 servings of grains, 5 servings of vegetables, 5 servings of fruits, 2 servings of milk and milk products, a maximum of 6 servings of lean meats, 4 servings of nuts and legume, and a maximum of 5 of sugars.

As per the serving sizes we provided earlier in this chapter, you have an exact idea of what type of grains you are allowed to eat and what amount makes one serving.

DASH Diet Exercise Routine

Everyone should follow some sort of exercise routine, whether suffering from a disease or healthy. Exercise is a must for those people who are suffering from some sort of disease; but in order to keep diseases at bay, healthy people are advised to also follow a moderate to light exercise regimen in order to ensure they stay healthy.

Keeping in mind, the fact that the DASH diet is designed for people who suffer from hypertension or those people who are expecting to lose weight, it is ideal that they remain active by exercising on a daily basis to gain the most benefit from this diet.

It is preferable that some sort of cardio routine is followed on at least 2-3 days in the week, and the rest of the days focusing toward strength training or body exercises be carried out. In order to stick to exercising, it is best if you start with any sport or activity that you personally enjoy. This is essential, due to the fact that if you enjoy an activity, there are higher chances that you will stick to it on a daily basis.

Beginners can start with a fifteen minute daily walk and then keep adding to it, as they are ready to increase intensity or duration.

Go Green Smoothie

Serves: 1

Ingredients

1 banana, peeled and sliced

1 cup packed with spinach leaves

Half cup of sliced mangoes

Half cup of milk, fat-free

Quarter cup of oats

Quarter cup of yogurt, fat-free

5 drops of vanilla essence

Recipe

Add banana, mango and oats to a blender and pour in yogurt. Blend until smooth, add milk, spinach and vanilla and blend again until the mixture reaches your desired consistency.

Enjoy!

Nutritious Breakfast Pudding

Serves: 4

Ingredients

One and a half cups of milk, fat-free

4 medium or large eggs

8 teaspoons of brown sugar

7 drops of vanilla essence

Half a teaspoon of cinnamon powder

Dash of salt

4 slices of diced whole wheat bread

1 apple, peeled and chopped finely

Quarter cup of raisins

Recipe

Preheat oven for fifteen minutes on a temperature of 350 degrees.

Prepare an 8 inch baking dish by coating it with butter.

Take a large mixing bowl, and add eggs and brown sugar.

Beat well for a minute.

Add in milk, cinnamon, salt and vanilla extract.

Whisk the mixture until a smooth paste is formed.

Mix in bread cubes, along with chopped apples and raisins.

Mix by folding the bread, apples and raisins in to the mixture and mix until bread looks soaked.

Spread the mixture into the prepared baking pan.

Cover the top of the dish with foil and place it in oven to bake for 35 minutes.

Bake uncovered for the next 20 minutes.

The pudding will have a golden color when it is ready.

Remove from oven and enjoy when slightly cooled.

Very Berry Smoothie

Serves: 4

Ingredients

2 cups of a mixture of your favorite berries, rinsed and sliced

1 cup of granola, low-fat

1 cup of yogurt, fat-free

Recipe

Add the berries into a blender and add in the yogurt. Blend till smooth.

Pour it into four glasses.

Top with the granola and sprinkle powdered sugar over the top.

Enjoy!

Power Packed Pancakes

Serves: 6

Ingredients

1 cup of milk, fat-free

1 cup of flour, whole wheat

Whites of 3 large eggs

1 large banana, peeled and sliced, then mashed

Quarter teaspoon of cinnamon

Dash salt

1 tablespoon oil

1 teaspoon baking powder

7 drops of vanilla essence

2 heaping tablespoons of your choice of dried fruits and nuts

Recipe

Take a large mixing bowl and add flour, salt, cinnamon and baking powder into it.

Mix well.

Add in eggs, one at a time, mixing after each addition.

Add in the milk and mix well.

Stir in mashed bananas, oil, and vanilla and mix well once again.

Fold in the dried fruit and nuts.

Heat a large pan and add a teaspoon of oil on to it.

Pour a quarter cup of the batter on to the pan. Do not disturb the pancake until bubbles start appearing on the surface.

Flip swiftly and let the other side cook, without pressing down on the pancake.

Remove and continue making pancakes out of the remaining batter.

Enjoy with low fat yogurt.

Healthy Oat Bread

Serves: 8

Ingredients

2 and half cups of uncooked oats

One third of a cup of sugar

One third of a cup of brown sugar

Dash of salt

3 and a quarter cups of milk, fat-free

2 large eggs

Half a tablespoon of vanilla extract

Recipe

Preheat oven for fifteen minutes on a temperature of 350 degrees.

Prepare an 8 inch baking dish by coating it with butter.

Take a large mixing bowl, and add oats and sugar.

Blend well for a minute, add salt and then mix again.

In another large bowl, combine milk and eggs.

Mix well, add vanilla extract and mix again.

Combine both mixtures together and mix until thoroughly combined.

Pour the oat mixture into the prepared dish.

Bake the mixture for 40 minutes, the center should come out wobbly.

Let cool slightly.

Take the brown sugar and sprinkle it over the baked oatmeal, until it is coating the top of the baked mixture in a thin layer.

Bake for a further 3 minutes until the sugar has melted.

Serve and Enjoy!

Peanut Butter Smoothie

Serves: 4

Ingredients

2 bananas, peeled and sliced

1 cup of milk, low-fat

1 tablespoon peanut butter, natural

Recipe

Add all the ingredients into the blender. Blend till smooth.

Enjoy!

French toast

Serves: 6

Ingredients

2 large eggs, beaten

Half cup of fat-free milk

1 teaspoon cinnamon powder

6 teaspoons of sugar

Quarter cup of natural applesauce

Slices of whole wheat bread

Recipe

Take a large mixing bowl and combine eggs and milk into it. Beat well.

Mix in cinnamon, applesauce and sugar. Mix well.

Dip each slice of bread into the mixture, and cook on a heated frying pan until golden brown.

Flip and fry the other side as well.

Remove and fry each of the remaining slices.

Serve and enjoy!

Tuna Salad

Serves: 2

Ingredients

Can of tuna in water

1 and a half tablespoons of olive oil

1 level tablespoon of vinegar, preferably red wine

2 cups of chopped tomatoes or whole cherry tomatoes

4 green onions, chopped

1 cup of cooked whole wheat pasta

Fresh parmesan cheese

Black pepper and salt to taste

Recipe

Take a large mixing bowl and add drained tuna to it. Mix in chopped green onions, tomatoes, pasta, and mix well. Pour oil, vinegar and sprinkle salt and pepper over the salad. Toss to coat.

Serve sprinkled with parmesan cheese!

DASH Pizza

Serves: 2

Ingredients

2 slices whole wheat regular bread, or pita bread

Half a cup, and slightly more, mozzarella cheese, low sodium

Quarter cup pizza sauce

Topping of choice can include, vegetables, corn, olives, mushrooms, bell pepper and chicken

Recipe

Preheat oven to 350 degrees.

If you are using bread, spread the sauce on it, but if you are using pita, then slice it open and spread the pizza sauce inside the pocket.

Add the toppings and cheese on the bread or inside the pocket of the pita bread.

Bake for 5 to 7 minutes until the bread or pita is toasted and the cheese is bubbling.

Serve hot and enjoy!

Pasta Salad

Serves: 4

Ingredients

4 cups pasta, whole wheat

1 cup Greek yogurt, low-fat or fat free

Quarter cup of chopped walnuts

1 teaspoon minced garlic

Quarter to one-third cup of mozzarella cheese, low-fat, low-sodium

Salt and Pepper

Quarter teaspoon of ground nutmeg

Half cup sun dried tomatoes

Quarter teaspoon olive oil

Recipe

Boil pasta until al dente, drain and reserve.

Place garlic and walnuts in a food processor along with cheese. Pulse mixture.

Add in yogurt and pepper, pulse until a smooth paste is formed.

Mix the ground paste into the pasta and mix well.

Drizzle olive oil on the salad and mix in tomatoes.

Ready to serve and enjoy!

Salad Skewers

Serves: 8

Ingredients

Half cup of bell peppers chopped into bite size pieces

Quarter cup of mushrooms chopped in bite size pieces

Quarter cup of tomatoes chopped in bite size pieces

Half cup of cucumbers chopped in bite size pieces

Half cup of spinach leaves chopped in bite size pieces

110 grams of cheddar cheese, low fat, sliced and further chopped

1 cup yogurt, low fat or fat free

2 tablespoons minced spring onion

30 ml of lime juice

Recipe

Take barbecue rods or skewers and place cubes of vegetables alternating with cheese.

In a large bowl combine the remaining ingredients to form a paste.

Apply the paste on the vegetable skewers using a brush.

Set in the refrigerator for 5 hours to cool and flavors to blend before serving.

Strawberry Salad

Serves: 8

Ingredients

6 tablespoons of olive oil

4 tablespoons of balsamic vinegar

4 tablespoons of water

Half a teaspoon of salt

Half a teaspoon of black pepper

1 onion, sliced

1 and a quarter pounds of prepared shrimp

4 cups of strawberries, sliced in quarters

16 cups of leafy green vegetables such as green lettuce, red lettuce, or kale, etc.

120 grams of feta cheese

2 medium cucumbers sliced or chopped

Recipe

Take a small bowl and mix together the first 5 ingredients.

Take another larger bowl and mix together the onions with 2 tablespoons of the prepared sauce.

Grill shrimp on a grill until they are done.

Take another 2 tablespoons of the sauce and coat strawberries in it.

Add salad greens and the onion mixture in another bowl with the remaining sauce, coat completely.

Divide the onion and leafy green mixture in eight servings and top with shrimp and strawberries.

Garnish with crumbled cheese and cucumbers.

Serve and Enjoy!

Walnut Salad

Serves: 4

Ingredients

Quarter cup of chopped toasted walnuts

1 cup of chopped apples

1 cup of chopped celery

Half a cup of dried fruits such as raisins or apricots

Quarter cup of yogurt

1 teaspoon icing sugar

8 ml of lemon juice

Recipe

Take a big bowl and combine chopped vegetables, fruits and dried fruits.

In a small bowl, mix yogurt, sugar and juice.

Toss the two mixtures together until thoroughly coated.

Serve and enjoy!

Wild Salad

Serves: 4

Ingredients

Half a teaspoon orange or lime zest

3 teaspoons balsamic vinegar

Salt to taste

Quarter cup of orange juice

One spring onion chopped finely

1 teaspoon mustard paste

Quarter cup of olive oil

3 cups of brown rice, cooked

1 cup of cherries, chopped

Half cup of dried fruit, such as cherries or apricots, etc.

Three-quarter cups of chopped celery

Quarter cup of toasted, chopped walnuts or pecans

Quarter cup of fresh, chopped parsley

120 grams of chopped cheddar cheese

Recipe

In a medium bowl, combine vinegar, salt, zest, mustard, olive oil, juice, and spring onion. Set aside. Mix in rice, dried fruits, cherries, celery, nuts, and parsley. Toss well. Top with cheese and serve.

Flavored Yogurt Cups

Serves: 4

Ingredients

Half a cup of shredded coconut

300 grams can of drained oranges or peaches in juice

1 sliced or diced banana

1 cup of sliced or diced strawberries

1 cup of diced or sliced mango

1 cup of yogurt, fat free or low fat

Recipe

Take a medium bowl and combine all the ingredients.

Serve and Enjoy!

Turkey Wraps

Serves: 4

Ingredients

1 whole wheat pita bread or pocketed bread

Mustard

Slices of smoked turkey, reduced sodium, reduced fat

1 pear or apple, sliced

Quarter cup of mozzarella cheese, low fat

Pepper and salt to taste

Recipe

Take bread and spread about a teaspoon of mustard inside it.

Place turkey slices in the pocket.

Add slices of fruits and sprinkle with salt, pepper and cheese.

Place in a toaster for a couple of minutes until cheese melts and fruit softens.

Serve and Enjoy!

Apple Muffins

Serves: 12

Ingredients

Three-quarters of a cup of flour

Three-quarters of a cup of whole wheat flour

2 teaspoons of cinnamon powder

1 teaspoon of baking powder

Half a teaspoon of baking soda

Dash of salt

1 cup of buttermilk, or 1 tablespoon of vinegar added to milk, fat free

Half a cup of oat bran

Quarter cup of brown sugar

6 teaspoons of vegetable oil

1 egg

4 apples, peeled, cored and chopped

Recipe

Preheat oven for 12 minutes at 400 degrees, and prepare a muffin pan by lining it with paper cups.

Take a large bowl and combine all the dry ingredients into it, including baking soda, baking powder, salt, flour and cinnamon.

In another bowl mix together buttermilk, oat bran, sugar, oil and egg.

Combine both of the mixtures and mix well.

Add in the apples and mix.

Pour the batter into the prepared pan.

Bake for 20 minutes until done. Test by inserting a toothpick into the center of one of the muffins, if it comes out clean it is done.

Serve and enjoy!

DASH Dip

Serves: 4

Ingredients

1 can of chickpeas, drained

1 cup of sour cream, fat free

2 teaspoons of garlic paste

5 tablespoons of balsamic vinegar

Quarter cup of tomatoes, sun dried

Quarter cup of chopped fresh parsley

3 tablespoons of chopped black olives

Recipe

Add all the ingredients in a food processor except tomatoes and olives. Blend until smooth.

Add in chopped tomatoes and olives.

Place the mix in a serving bowl and garnish with olives. Serve with assorted vegetables and crackers for dipping.

DASH Blueberry Muffins

Serves: 12

Ingredients

One and a half cups of flour

Half cup of whole wheat flour

Half teaspoon of baking powder

Quarter teaspoon of baking soda

Dash of salt

1 cup of milk

Half a cup of milk powder, fat-free

One third of a cup of sugar

6 teaspoons of vegetable oil

1 egg

1 cup of blueberries

Recipe

Preheat oven for 12 minutes at 400 degrees, and prepare a muffin pan by lining it with paper cups.

Take a large bowl and combine all the dry ingredients into it, including baking soda, baking powder, dry milk, salt and flour.

In another bowl mix together milk, sugar, oil and egg.

Combine both of the mixtures and mix well.

Add in the blueberries and mix.

Pour the batter into the prepared pan.

Bake for 20 minutes until done. Test by inserting a toothpick into the center of one of the muffins, if it comes out clean it is done.

Serve and enjoy!

Paradise in a Cup Smoothie

Serves: 3

Ingredients

2 cups of melon or cantaloupe, chopped

1 cup of flavored tangy yogurt, low fat

1 cup of orange juice

Recipe

Add all the ingredients to a blender and process until smooth.

Pour into glasses and enjoy!

DASH Hummus

Serves: 3

Ingredients

One-third of a cup of tahini

One-eighth of a teaspoon of red chili flakes

2 cups of canned chickpeas

One-eighth of a teaspoon of lemon juice

Half a teaspoon of minced garlic

Salt and pepper to taste

2 tablespoons of olive oil

Recipe

Add chickpeas, chili, garlic, tahini, salt, pepper, juice and blend well until smooth.

Mix in the oil.

Spoon in to a bowl, and leave for an hour to let the flavors blend together.

Serve as a dip.

Oat Muffins

Serves: 8

Ingredients

1 and three quarters cup of old fashioned oats

8 teaspoons of brown sugar

1 cup plus 2 tablespoons of flour

Half a cup of sugar

1 tablespoon of baking powder

Dash of salt

1 cup of milk, low-fat or fat free

1 egg

2 tablespoons of oil

1 teaspoon lemon or orange zest

1 teaspoon of vanilla essence

Recipe

Preheat oven for 12 minutes at 400 degrees, and prepare a muffin pan by lining it with paper cups.

Take a large bowl and combine all the dry ingredients into it, including baking powder, salt, zest, sugar, (one and a half cup) oats and flour.

In another bowl mix together milk, vanilla, oil and egg.

Combine both of the mixtures and mix well.

In a small bowl, combine remaining quarter cup of oats with brown sugar and mix.

Pour the batter into the prepared pan.

Top with oat and brown sugar mixture.

Bake for 20 minutes until done. Test by inserting a toothpick into the center of one of the muffins, if it comes out clean it is done.

Serve and enjoy.

Lemon Buttermilk

Serves: 3

Ingredients

Half a cup of cold milk, fat-free or low-fat

180 grams of yogurt, low-fat

2 tablespoons sugar

1 teaspoon of lemon juice

Half a teaspoon of lemon or lime zest

Recipe

Combine all the ingredients together in a blender jug.

Blend together until smooth.

Serve in glasses and enjoy!

DASH Dinner

Chicken Dinner

Serves: 8

Ingredients

1 cup of orange juice

2 tablespoons of soy sauce, reduced sodium

2 tablespoons of szechuan sauce

1 and a half tablespoons of cornstarch

1 tablespoon of oil

2 pounds of chicken breast, chopped into cube size pieces

4 cups of broccoli

300 grams of peas

4 cups of cabbage, chopped or shredded

4 cups of brown rice

2 tablespoons of sesame seeds

Recipe

In a medium sized bowl, combine juice, sauces and cornstarch.

Take a pan or a wok, and heat oil in it. Add the cubed chicken and stir fry until done, approximately 7 to 10 minutes.

Add broccoli, cabbage, peas and the sauces. Mix well and stir fry for another 5 to 8 minutes. Add in seeds and serve with cooked brown rice.

Beef in Grilled Pineapple

Serves: 12

Ingredients

3 pounds of beef, cut in to bite sized pieces

Salt and pepper, for rubbing on beef

4 tablespoons of lemon juice

5 tablespoons of oil

3 teaspoons of minced garlic

3 jalapeno, chopped

1 teaspoon cumin powder

6 cups pineapple chunks

2 onions, chopped into cubes

2 bell pepper, chopped into cubes

4 teaspoons of lemon or lime zest

1 teaspoon of salt

Recipe

Rub the chopped beef with salt and pepper.

In a medium sized bowl, combine lemon juice, oil, garlic, jalapenos and cumin powder. Mix well.

Reserve 4 tablespoons of the mixture, rub the rest of it on the beef and keep it aside for 2 hours.

Remove the beef and start threading it on skewers alternating with chopped vegetables pieces.

Place skewers on grill and cook for 15 minutes until beef is done and vegetables softened, and coat with the reserved marinade each time the skewers are turned.

Serve and enjoy.

Sausage and Beans

Serves: 6

Ingredients

1 tablespoon of oil

250 grams of sausages, chopped

1 cup chopped onions

1 teaspoon of minced garlic

1 bell pepper, chopped

Half a tablespoon of cumin powder

1 cup brown rice, uncooked

400 grams of canned beans

500 ml of water

Recipe

Take a skillet or sauce pan and heat oil in it.

Fry onions and sausages, until onions turn transparent.

Add in vegetables, rice, beans and seasonings. Mix well.

Add in water and let it boil.

Once boiled, let the pot simmer for 30 to 40 minutes until rice is cooked through.

Serve and Enjoy!

Tangy Halibut

Serves: 3

Ingredients

Half a kilo of Halibut fillets

1 cup yogurt

1 teaspoon of minced garlic

Quarter teaspoon of pepper

Quarter teaspoon of lemon juice

Quarter teaspoon of salt

Recipe

In a small bowl combine lemon juice, garlic, seasonings and yogurt and stir well.

Take a grill pan or frying pan and grill or fry fillets on both sides until done.

Add the sauce on top of the fish and let it cook in the sauce for two minutes more.

Serve warm and enjoy!

Chili Stir Fry

Serves: 3

Ingredients

1 kilo of squash

500 grams of chili peppers

2 tablespoons of oil

1 cup chopped onion

1 teaspoon pepper and salt

Chili powder to taste

1 cup of any cheese, grated

Recipe

Prepare the squash by coring, de-seeding, peeling and chopping it into cubes.

Roast chilies on stove top, until charred.

Once cooled, de-seed and chop the chilies

Take a sauce pan and heat oil in it.

Add onions and cook until transparent.

Add the squash and seasonings to the pot.

Place the lid on and let cook for 15 minutes, while stirring occasionally.

Add in the chopped chilies and cook for additional 5 minutes.

Add in cheese and cover until melted.

Serve and enjoy!

Orange Chicken

Serves: 4

Ingredients

1 cup yogurt

Half a cup of onion, minced

2 tablespoons of cilantro, diced

1 tablespoon of honey

Salt to taste

Black pepper to taste

4 to 5, 150 grams chicken breasts

1 ripe avocado

Quarter cup of lemon or lime juice

2 oranges, chopped

1 onion, sliced

Recipe

Take a bowl and mix in yogurt, minced onions, honey, cilantro, black pepper and salt.

Mix well.

Coat the mixture on the chicken thoroughly.

Leave the marinade on the chicken for 30 minutes.

Grill the chicken until done.

In another bowl, add chopped and peeled avocado. Pour in the lemon juice and coat well.

Mix in oranges and onions.

When chicken is done, serve with the onion and avocado mixture on the side.

Enjoy!

Cocoa Pudding

Serves: 8

Ingredients

6 tablespoons of corn flour

4 tablespoons of unsweetened dark cocoa powder

4 tablespoons of sugar, grinded

Dash and bit more of salt

1 liter of milk, low fat

Half a cup of semi sweet chocolate chips

1 teaspoon of vanilla essence

Recipe

In a saucepan, add corn flour, sugar, cocoa powder and salt. Mix well.

Pour in milk and mix well.

Over medium heat, cook the mixture until thickened, stirring constantly to keep from burning.

Once it reaches desired consistency, stir in chocolate chips and essence. Mix well.

Serve and enjoy!

Walnut and Chocolate Cookies

Serves: 20

Ingredients

2 cups of old fashioned oats

Half a cup of flour

Half a cup of whole-wheat flour

1 teaspoon of cinnamon powder

Half a teaspoon of baking soda

Half a teaspoon of salt

Half a cup of sesame sauce (tahini)

Quarter cup of cold cubed butter

Two-third of a cup of sugar

Two-third of a cup of brown sugar

1 egg

1 egg white

1 teaspoon vanilla essence

1 cup of chocolate chips

Half a cup of chopped walnuts

Recipe

Preheat oven to 350 degrees.

Prepare two cookie sheets by lining with butter paper.

In a medium bowl, add oats, flours, baking soda, cinnamon and salt and mix well.

In another bowl combine cold cubed butter with tahini and beat well on medium speed with an electric beater, until thoroughly incorporated.

In the same bowl, mix in brown sugar and white sugar, continue beating with electric beater on medium speed, until smooth.

Add in whole egg, vanilla, and egg white. Continue beating until combined.

To this mixture, add the oat mixture and mix well.

Fold in the nuts and chocolate.

With slightly moist hands, start rolling teaspoonfuls of the mixture into balls.

Place the balls on cookie sheet, 2 inches apart and flatten slightly by pressing with the back of a spoon lightly.

Place the cookie sheets in the oven and bake for 15 minutes, until golden brown in color.

Let cool before serving or they might break on being moved too soon.

Popsicles

Serves: 12

Ingredients

2 cups of chopped blueberries

2 cups of chopped blackberries

2 cups of yogurt, fat-free or low-fat

2 and a half cups of milk, fat-free or low-fat

Recipe

Add the berries into a blender and add in the yogurt. Blend until smooth.

Pour in the milk and blend once again.

Pour into moulds or cups.

Place in a freezer for about twenty minutes.

After twenty minutes, insert sticks into the moulds and let freeze for several hours until completely hard.

Remove from freezer when it's time to serve and enjoy!

Blackberry Mock

Serves: 8

Ingredients

6 teaspoons of sugar

3 teaspoons of corn flour

2 cups of chopped blackberries

Half a teaspoon of lemon juice

Half a cup of oats

Quarter cup of flour

Quarter cup of brown sugar

2 pinches ground cinnamon

Dash of salt

3 teaspoons of butter, unsalted

Quarter cup of chopped walnuts or hazelnuts

Recipe

Preheat oven for 12 minutes at 400 degrees, and prepare a baking pan by coating it with cooking spray.

Take a medium sized bowl and incorporate sugar and corn flour until thoroughly combined. Mix in the berries and juice. Stir well to combine all the ingredients.

Pour the mixture into the prepared pan.

Clean and wipe the same mixing bowl, and into this bowl, add oats, brown sugar, salt, cinnamon and flour. Mix well.

Add in to this mixture, the butter and blend with a fork until mixture is crumbly.

Mix in the nuts. Add this oat topping to the berry mixture. Do not mix.

Bake for 30 minutes and serve after cooling for 10 minutes.

Berry Crumble

Serves: 8

Ingredients

3 cups of chopped strawberries, blueberries and blackberries

3 teaspoons of diced softened butter, unsalted

3 teaspoons of all purpose flour

3 teaspoons of brown sugar

Half a cup of oats

2 pinches of ground cinnamon

Recipe

Preheat oven for 12 minutes at 400 degrees, and prepare a pie pan by coating it with cooking spray.

In a medium sized bowl, combine all the ingredients apart from the berries and mix well.

Add the washed and dried berries to the pie pan and top it with the oat mixture. Do not mix.

Bake for 30 minutes and serve after cooling for 10 minutes.

Quick and Healthy Trifle

Serves: 8

Ingredients

2 pears, peeled and sliced

6 teaspoons of lemon juice

2 cups of chopped strawberries

7 drops of almond extract or vanilla

6 teaspoons of orange juice

6 teaspoons of honey

Small cake cubes

3 cups of flavored yogurt

Recipe

Place fruits in a medium sized bowl and pour lemon juice on top of it along with extract. Toss well.

In a smaller bowl, mix together orange juice and honey.

Take a glass dish and start creating layers by placing about a third of the cake cubes first, then pour a tablespoon of the orange and honey mixture on the cubes.

Pour a cup of the flavored yogurt next, followed by a cup of each of the fruits.

Repeat this procedure to create two more layers.

Refrigerate for 4 to 5 hours.

Serve!

DASH Diet & Day Meal Planner

The DASH Diet allows three meals and two snacks in a day. There is no fixed rule as to what you should eat on any of these days. You can choose any of the breakfast recipes from the recipes given. Same goes for lunch, dinner and snacks. Follow any of the recipes you like and repeat it as many times as you want.

However you must remain within the allowed food and serving sizes in order to achieve the maximum benefits from the DASH Diet.

Crucial DASH Diet Tips

1. If you work for 8 hours a day, and you don't have time to prepare meals, you can always purchase cut up vegetables from grocery stores and salad bars. However stay away from the dressings and fattening salads.

2. You could also purchase frozen vegetables as they are very convenient to use and easy to prepare.

3. Add berries into your diet, as it will cover your daily requirement for fruits in a delicious and easy way.

4. Mix low-fat yogurt with berries and nuts for a quick, healthy and delicious snack to revive you during a workday.

5. Eat nuts salt free.

6. Add smoothies to your diet, to gain benefit from healthy fruits and vegetables.

7. Make exercising a regular part of your diet.